THE POWER TO PIVOT

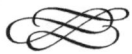

HELEN RHODES, MD

ISBN eBook: 979-8-9927257-1-1

ISBN paperback: 979-8-9927257-0-4

ISBN hardcover: 979-8-9927257-2-8

To my daughters
Whose best interests have always been central to the career decisions
I've made
You are my heart

CONTENTS

INTRODUCTION: LEARNING TO PIVOT

My goal in writing this book is to help other physicians move beyond feelings of disillusionment and frustration at whatever point they may be in their careers so they can thrive. The current generation of doctors is working and learning within a medical system that is very different from the one I trained in over thirty years ago, and their struggles are even more complex. They must overcome financial insecurity due to large educational debt, balance a demanding career with caring for their children, and grapple with the erosion of physician autonomy when employed by a large healthcare system.

Our healthcare structure has become corporatized, putting profit before people. The inordinate amount of time spent on administrative tasks, such as electronic health record (EHR) documentation and coding, is designed solely to maximize revenue for commercial entities. These organizations usurp physicians' autonomy and compromise the once-sacred doctor-patient relationship. It does not improve quality of care and it significantly contributes to the rising number of physicians experiencing burnout. Unfortunately, burnout is occurring earlier in a doctor's career trajectory, leading some to choose early retirement.

Physicians are feeling *frustrated* by the time required to complete clerical details that take them away from patient care, *angry* over the declining payments from insurance companies, *betrayed* by those who do not have their best interests at heart, and *saddened* by the growing mistrust of the medical community by the American people in a system that is no longer designed to benefit them. This leads to grievous moral injury. It is imperative to keep the United States medical workforce robust given the current physician shortage and growing demand for the care of patients with chronic complex medical conditions.

Despite these pessimistic realities, applications to medical schools in the US remain at an all-time high and continue to increase, which indicates that becoming a part of our noble profession is still coveted.

Career options for newly minted physicians include academics, hospitalist work, locum tenens, and multispecialty group or private practice. Sadly, even though the option of going solo provides the most autonomy, fewer are choosing this path. The declining reimbursements from insurance companies and rising costs of running a business make this choice less attractive and not financially feasible. Most young doctors choose employed positions upon completion of residency and/or fellowship training.

I've been fortunate to have worked in a variety of settings including academics, private practice, full-time, part-time, and not at all. Currently, I blend ownership of a solo gynecology practice with locum tenens work. This has allowed me to experience professional fulfillment and a "career renaissance."

I hope that the story of my professional journey with its stops and starts, and successes and failures, will inspire other physicians and help them move past feelings of disillusionment, frustration, financial insecurity, and powerlessness. By learning from my experiences, I want my colleagues, especially those who are younger, to be empowered to choose the paths that lead to better work-life balance, professional fulfillment, and eventual longevity in their chosen specialties.

In 2013, uncertainty rippled through my professional and personal life.

There had been recent leadership changes at the cancer center where I held an academic position, and I felt as though I was purposefully being left out of important departmental and institutional decisions. My mentor had resigned from the institution and my section chief, whom I once considered a friend, became more distant, leading to my feelings of betrayal. I felt as though my ideas and efforts were being brushed aside, and I had a target on my back due to undeserved negative feedback I had received at my annual review.

I was a single mom and experiencing financial stress as my eldest daughters, Jane and Sarah, were in college, and my youngest daughter Maggie was finishing her last years in high school.

I was walking on eggshells.

I needed to learn how to *pivot*.

During this challenging time, Wilson entered my life. I met him through mutual friends and was instantly captivated by his handsomeness and warm, easy conversation. We started dating, and he reintroduced me to the wonders of the Texas coast that I had enjoyed so much as a child. We began spending time sailing on Galveston Bay.

Although I had briefly learned the basics of sailing in middle school, for Wilson, it was a lifelong hobby. He enthusiastically shared his passion for the sea, showing me the ropes and teaching me the intricacies of what may appear to some as an easy pastime. Because I wanted to impress him and not run his boat aground or fall overboard, I spent time earnestly reading the books he had given me. I discovered that the nuances of learning to sail could be as challenging as mastering the steps taken in the operating room to complete complex laparoscopic surgery.

Sailing on Galveston Bay provided an unexpected yet necessary diversion from my real world.

On a day in the early fall, when we had decided to take his boat out into the bay, the breeze was southerly with an easterly component. I had learned to read the wind direction by looking at the flags flying high atop the flagpoles in the marina. I was positioned at the helm, while one other crew member, Colin, was first mate.

To get out of the marina through the dredged channel aligned by red and green markers and into the bay, it was necessary to keep the diesel engine running while I steered, and the crew readied the sails. This journey from the marina past the restaurants and amusement park rides of the boardwalk into the bay always seemed to take longer than it really was.

A necessary lesson in patience.

"What's your course?" Wilson asked as the boat passed through the last red and green channel markers.

"I'm feeling the wind on the right side of my face, so let's head into the wind," I answered.

I gave the commands to tack the boat as I had been taught and done so many times before.

"Ready about?" followed by, "Hard a lee!"

In response to the crew's reply of "Ready!"

I then maneuvered the boat's bow into the wind as the men hoisted the main sail.

"Fall off!" Wilson shouted.

As I slightly changed the direction of the bow, the majestic main sail above me filled quickly becoming taut with a pop, akin to a sheet tied to a clothesline getting its wrinkles puffed out by the wind.

Wilson turned off the engine and, in an instant, complete tranquility ensued, accompanied by the soft lapping sounds of the small waves in the bay, tweets of the birds flying above, and the gentle breeze flowing against my cheeks.

A thirty-five-foot-eight-ton vessel completely powered by the wind. Such a spectacular feat of physics combined with skill, a checklist, and trust.

The parallels of sailing to decisions regarding my professional life have become clearer over the past decade.

The professional autonomy and fulfillment I have achieved impart the same feelings of accomplishment I get when powering a sailboat using only the wind.

The components of the vessel, along with the well-thought-out sailing plan are all integral parts of a system that ultimately leads to the goal of moving freely in an environment of solitude and peace. And the direction of the wind, position of the rudder, and angle of the sails are vectors that can affect the boat's course. A crew must be able to pivot quickly when one or more of these changes, and likewise, I've found that I need to pivot quickly when my professional circumstances change.

Since choosing obstetrics and gynecology (Ob/Gyn) as my specialty over thirty years ago, I have endured external forces that were often out of my control, and I have had to adapt when these unexpected changes occurred.

Through a lengthy, iterative process that has followed a sinuous course, I ultimately arrived at a point of peace by blending ownership of a solo micro practice with locum tenens work. These additional jobs, commonly referred to as "side gigs," have helped me remain financially secure when the revenue from my practice wasn't optimal. Thus, I feel it is possible to be fulfilled as a solo private practice physician as well as financially secure by building a career portfolio.

There wasn't a playbook for this journey, and I am indebted to the many people who cheered me on, inspired me, and even panned me along the way.

As you read my story, I encourage you to reflect on what changes you might consider making in your current career situation that will satisfy your heart while maintaining your autonomy.

THE BEGINNING—EARLY INFLUENCES

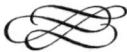

For most of us, the desire to pursue a career in medicine is deeply rooted in our childhood and young adult experiences. My decision to go to medical school was greatly influenced by my relationship with my grandmother, the support of my parents, and my love of science.

My grandparents graduated from medical school in Scotland in the 1920s and practiced in Liverpool, England until they retired. Because my family immigrated from the UK to the US in 1966 when I was almost four, I didn't get to spend much time with them. After my grandfather died in the 1970s, my grandmother moved to Texas and lived in an apartment close by.

My four siblings and I would take turns spending the night at Grandma's. She spoiled us by indulging us with our favorite meals and television programs. When it was my turn, I looked forward to a menu of baked white fish with dill sauce and fluffy mashed potatoes. For dessert, I savored meringue casings filled with homemade strawberry ice cream topped with fresh berries and whipped cream. We sat outside on her small balcony for meals where I was captivated by my grandmother's stories of practicing medicine in Liverpool during The Blitz as well as taking care of her pediatric patients before the discovery of penicillin. How I wish I had written more of her stories down!

After dinner, the television program lineup included *The Mary Tyler Moore Show* and *The Carol Burnett Show*. I only pretended to be interested in the articles from *The British Medical Journal* that Grandma had dog-eared for me to read. Reading them, however, did help me to fall asleep in my sleeping bag on her living room floor.

Grandma's energy was amazing. She loved to race up the stairs to her third-floor apartment and insisted on getting "brown" in the Texas sun while sipping hot tea with milk by her apartment complex's swimming pool. She loved Blue Bell vanilla ice cream, Jimmy Carter, the Dallas Cowboys, and the Texas Longhorns.

For five years, we were treated to special times with our grandmother. I was quite sad when she moved back to the UK. Her reasons involved her pension, health insurance, and Medicare. She believed that access to healthcare was a right, not a privilege.

Looking back, I realize that Grandma was my first mentor.

As a child, I was fascinated by science and the intricacies of the human body, which was further fueled by my mother's career in nursing. Mom easily juggled work and volunteer commitments with taking care of our family. I marvel now at her amazing mothering of the five of us. She volunteered for the March of Dimes and brought home an illustrated atlas, which contained descriptions of genetic defects that could occur during pregnancy. I was completely fascinated by the contents of this book, along with another one called *Being Born,* which described the development of a baby from fertilization to birth. I was mesmerized by its contents and would hide the book under my bedcovers to read after "lights out" had been declared by my parents.

My father is a retired physicist who studied at Cambridge University. We moved to Austin in 1966 for his job as a project manager for a private corporation whose work was funded by the US Atomic Energy Commission. The five of us enjoyed visiting his office and laboratory, where experiments focusing on the use of x-ray energy were being conducted. I was fascinated by the oversized canister of liquid nitrogen in one of the labs as well as the enormous periodic table pinned to one of the walls in his office. I spent one summer as a teen working with Dad and his post-doctoral scientist on experiments designed to calibrate the concentration of chloride ions in concrete.

Dad was always tinkering. Fixing broken things around the house, putting soles back onto his shoes with Shoe Goo, and building model airplanes with my brothers. He spent time on the weekends teaching me how everything worked in the engine of my first car, a Triumph Spitfire. I purchased that little sports vehicle with money I had earned from babysitting and working at the bowling alley. The car had a stick shift, and Dad patiently taught me how to drive it in the parking lot of my high school.

My plan was to enter college as a biology pre-med major, which was the script at the time for those of us interested in going to medical school. However, I received an unexpected invitation to be a part of the freshman engineering honors program at my chosen university, which came with a small scholarship. I really didn't want to be an engineer, but with my parents' encouragement, I accepted.

During college, I juggled a rigorous course schedule while participating in sorority and other social activities. I also worked at various part-time jobs to help pay for my tuition and living expenses. Despite changing my degree plan during my third year and not having enough course credits to graduate, I was accepted into medical school following the completion of my senior year.

During the third year of medical school, I was one of those students who thoroughly enjoyed each rotation, declaring, "This is it" every time I started a new one. I was particularly drawn to surgery. My experience as a patient when I ruptured my eardrum in a water-skiing accident in college prompted me to select otolaryngology for residency training, hoping to eventually be a plastic surgeon. At that time, otolaryngology residency acceptances were awarded ahead of the regular match.

I had purposely placed Ob/Gyn near the end of my third-year clinical rotation schedule because I absolutely knew I wouldn't select this specialty. The lifestyle was felt to be exceptionally difficult due to the hours of obstetrical night call and the potential for malpractice lawsuits.

I was sitting in a lecture with our small group of about a dozen students, including one of my closest friends. We had both decided we were not going to consider a career in Ob/Gyn. I was intently listening to the lecture when my friend began kicking me under the table, elbowing me, and whispering, "I really like this. I thought we said that we weren't going to do this?"

I giggled, as I was feeling the same way.

By then, I had completed my applications for an otolaryngology residency and was preparing to set up interviews. Otolaryngology, Ob/Gyn, ophthalmology, and orthopedic surgery were part of the "O" collection that were considered to be more competitive programs.

I was drawn to Ob/Gyn because of the opportunity to take care of women of all ages during many different phases of their lives. From delivering babies to helping women navigate changes associated with menopause, this specialty combines the disciplines of surgery and medicine. The surgeries span everything from a simple dilatation and curettage (D&C) to complex staging procedures for gynecologic cancers.

I remember learning to deliver a baby using the "football maneuver," scrubbing in to assist during hysterectomies, and absorbing endocrinology lectures given by our department chair, who taught me about "all things hormonal." The *pièce de résistance* was when I was allowed to do my first minor surgical procedure as the primary surgeon under the guidance of my attending physician.

Ob/Gyn was fun. The patients were generally healthy, not suffering from chronic diseases, and they didn't die. This was important to me as I felt significant emotional and visceral discomfort when involved with the care of terminal patients.

After the lecture when I experienced the "aha moment" with my classmate, I stopped the application process for otolaryngology and began pursuing the next steps for a residency in obstetrics and gynecology.

During my fourth year, I spent two months in Houston. It was

1987, and there were three Ob/Gyn residency programs in the city. I spent one month on the maternal-fetal medicine service at one and the second month on the gynecology-pathology service at another.

I loved hobnobbing with the residents and hearing their stories of why they picked the programs they were training in, and what their eventual career plans were.

It was a joyful time. The days and weeks ran together as I totally immersed myself in my chosen specialty and fell in love with it. Each day brought me closer to the reality that this was the right decision for me despite what my medical school friend and I had decided we were *not* going to pursue.

On match day, I opened the envelope to read that I had been selected by my first choice residency program.

I was ecstatic and eager to get started.

- *When life is challenging, take the time to reflect on early positive influences so that you can become realigned with your purpose.*
- *Don't ever forget why you chose the specialty you chose.*
- *When disillusioned, reflect on the mentors who inspired you to become a physician.*

RESIDENCY AND FIRST JOB

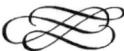

*T*here's something cruel and nonsensical about the transition from being a medical school graduate to becoming an intern. From being on top of the world to trying to swim in quicksand, I worried that my knowledge and skillset were inadequate. The sleep deprivation and almost complete loss of my personal life afforded no time for self-care and took their toll. Days blurred from one to the next.

I feel that regardless of which residency a physician selects, whether it is a competitive academic program or an "easier" community-based program, the feelings of completely plummeting are the same.

Unfortunately, not much has changed since the years I was a resident. It's exhausting. That distinctive feeling of having toothpicks in your eyes, scratchy unbathed skin, and wondering when you last ate or brushed your teeth are universal.

During my residency training, I decided to pursue a fellowship in maternal-fetal medicine. My decision was influenced by my chairman and so many of the faculty who are world-renowned specialists in this field.

But pivoting is sometimes necessary to achieve the work-life balance we crave and deserve.

After starting the application process for the fellowship, two things happened almost simultaneously.

First, I learned I was pregnant with my eldest daughter Jane, and second, I rotated on the gynecology surgery service, where I began performing complex gynecologic procedures as the primary surgeon. This included an assignment at the cancer center, where I was placed on the oncology team. While I felt that caring for cancer patients was extremely challenging, I enjoyed the surgical aspect of this rotation. The more surgeries I learned how to do, the more I realized how much I loved being in the operating room. I didn't want to give up this part of my skill set, which I felt would happen as a maternal-fetal medicine specialist.

In 1992, academic medicine, multispecialty group practice, fellowship training, and private practice were the choices for jobs upon completion of Ob/Gyn training. I was afraid that juggling the care of a new baby along with any of these options would be beyond what I was capable of, and I had a difficult time deciding.

Before I found an adequate solution, an unexpected job opportunity materialized.

On the gynecologic oncology service at the cancer center, I worked with an inspirational, brilliant, and entrepreneurial physician. Her vision was to open a cancer screening and detection clinic at the institution. She created a general gynecology position and offered me the job. Subsequently, she became my mentor.

The job description appealed to me for several reasons. The hours would be Monday through Friday without night call or weekend responsibilities, which meant I could spend more time at home with my daughter Jane. And I would have the opportunity to work with residents and fellows, receive strong mentoring, be involved with research projects, and perform a lot of surgeries.

I accepted the position without hesitation, and thus my academic career began. My mentor wanted me to start my new job just two days after our graduation gala. All my residency colleagues were taking a few months off before beginning their first jobs and had looked at several options before signing on the dotted line.

Not me. I plunged right in.

Because I had chosen a gynecology-only position right out of training, I needed to plan a way to collect obstetrical cases for my oral board examination, which I would be eligible for after completing the first two years of employment. The oral board exam required that the case list include both obstetrics and gynecology.

I was able to negotiate a volunteer night call opportunity in Labor and Delivery (L&D) at the institution where I had completed my residency. This allowed me to collect the requisite Ob cases for my oral boards. Instead of compensation, my medical liability (medmal) insurance coverage was paid for by my department.

I enjoyed returning to the institution where I had trained, working with the junior residents, as well as the opportunity to maintain my skill set.

My schedule at the cancer center included seeing patients in the outpatient clinic, operating, teaching, and participating in clinical research projects. This is the proverbial "three-legged stool" of academic medicine consisting of clinical work, teaching, and research. All three legs are necessary to achieve promotion and tenure.

Despite the seemingly easy schedule compared to that of my colleagues, who were taking night call and working on weekends, I found the combination of a full-time academic position and taking care of a toddler too challenging, and I negotiated a part-time position during the second year of my contract.

Shortly after the approval of a part-time position, I became pregnant with my second daughter, Sarah. Unfortunately, I developed complications during my pregnancy and was placed on bed rest for several months. It was the early 1990s, before the development of the internet, and I was unable to do much of anything. I relied on my nanny, Betsy, to care for Jane while I lay in bed. I filled the long boring days of bedrest by ordering Christmas presents from mail order catalogs, reading medical journals, and writing an academic paper.

After Sarah was born and I returned to work, I realized that the pressures of academic medicine were too much for me to blend with my desire to have more children and be at home. Even though I was taking a few L&D night call shifts each month, I missed taking care of obstetrical patients in the outpatient setting. I left the cancer center six months after Sarah's birth and began looking for new opportunities.

This would be the first of two instances in which I completely left medical practice.

- *My hope is that positive changes regarding career options will occur for the younger generation of physicians in training so that they do not become disillusioned and burned out as quickly as is currently happening.*
- *Some opportunities drop into our lives and others we must create.*
- *I highly recommend keeping your clinical skills current throughout your career, even when on sabbatical or working in a non-clinical role. If you ever decide to return to direct patient care after a hiatus, most employers require documentation of clinical proficiency in your specialty.*

FIRST CAREER PIVOT LEADING TO SECOND JOB

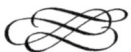

*M*y current career situation, that of blending ownership of a gynecology micro practice with Ob/Gyn locum tenens jobs, was not by design. Rather, it is the cumulation of decades of transitioning through different professional opportunities and pivoting when a position no longer aligned with my personal and professional goals. I feel it merits a discussion of the timeline of my career to better understand each work situation as it applied to my personal life at the time, as well as why I made the decisions I made to transition to a different opportunity.

There isn't a playbook for our lives. Learning to recognize when our personal and professional goals are out of alignment is crucial to becoming empowered to leave a less-than-ideal situation in search of something better.

Don't be afraid to pivot. Don't be afraid to step outside the box when examining professional opportunities that present themselves.

Dig deep and dig often.

* * *

AFTER LEAVING THE CANCER CENTER, I filled my days with caring for my daughters. Jane had started preschool while Sarah was still an infant. I loved dropping my older girl off and picking her up, scheduling playdates and outings to the park, menu planning, grocery shopping, and being "domestic".

Just as I had seen my mother do.

While Jane was at her program and Sarah was napping, I began researching opportunities for my next job. I considered the option of starting a solo private practice. I painstakingly listed every supply I would need in my exam rooms, right down to the number of cotton balls. I met with the Chief Executive Officer (CEO) of a local hospital to inquire about leasing office space and the possibility of financial support in the form of an income guarantee.

It didn't take me long to realize that the logistics of opening a private practice were daunting.

I abandoned the idea of starting a new practice and continued to search job boards and ultimately discovered a posting for an Ob/Gyn position with a multispecialty group practice. The organization had clinics all over the Houston area with centralized hospital care for maternity and surgical patients. The clinic that had the opening was located thirty minutes from our home, while the hospital was thirty minutes away in the opposite direction.

I interviewed for the position and learned I would be working alongside a women's health nurse practitioner. Ella possessed a delightful personality and made me feel instantly welcome. I discovered she had a part-time schedule, so I inquired if this would be a possibility for me. I was thrilled when my request was granted.

Between us, Ella and I would cover all the clinic days. She would see the low-risk obstetrical patients, perform routine Gyn exams, provide birth control counseling, and manage minor gynecologic complaints. I would be available for physician consultation for patients who she felt might benefit from surgical intervention or who had high-risk obstetrical conditions.

We made a great team and became close friends in addition to being colleagues. I learned so much from Ella regarding the care of Ob/Gyn patients in a community setting.

My contract was for sixty percent of a full-time position, which equaled three days per week. On Monday, I would operate in the morning at the centralized hospital location and see patients at the suburban office in the afternoon. I would see a full day of patients on Tuesday and Thursday and be off on Wednesday and Friday, which gave me lots of time to be with my daughters. Ella saw patients on Tuesday, Wednesday, and Friday, giving us one day in the office together when I could assist with physician consultations. I also saw patients one Saturday morning each month for women who were unable to make appointments during the week.

My call schedule was also part-time, consisting of three call shifts per month. We were in-house for twenty-four hours with the next day off. Interestingly, this hospitalist model of care was not formalized throughout the country until twenty years later. Our group worked at several clinic locations, and we set up subgroups to handle hospital rounding responsibilities so that not everyone was required to go to the hospital each day.

The position afforded a nice work-life balance and demonstrated that it is possible to work part-time and take excellent care of patients by partnering with a nurse practitioner and utilizing a centralized hospitalist model of care. It was 1995, and this employment model for Ob/Gyns was ahead of its time.

In addition to my clinical responsibilities, I learned the basics of coding and billing, joined committees, and wrote practice guidelines for our group. These activities kept my academic brain stimulated.

I was happy with the work-life balance. It allowed me to take care of a small volume of obstetrical patients and perform surgeries with coverage for hospital rounds and clinic on the days I was off.

My third daughter Maggie was born a year later, and when she was eighteen months old, I became pregnant with my fourth child.

I felt I had achieved a nearly perfect work-life balance and truly felt this position would be my forever job.

Then, tragedy struck.

ENDURING TRAGEDY AND ITS AFTERMATH

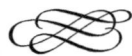

$\mathscr{I}$t was the Saturday before Christmas, and I was on call. My sister Sam, who was also pregnant and due a few weeks after me, was out shopping with her husband. They were planning to visit his parents for the holidays and asked if I could do an ultrasound to determine their baby's sex.

It wasn't very busy at the hospital, so I excitedly invited Sam and my brother-in-law to come. I was not able to determine with certainty what she was having, but felt like the baby was likely a boy. After I finished scanning my sister, she wanted to look at my baby, so I proceeded to perform an ultrasound on myself.

My baby's heart wasn't beating.

I was twenty weeks.

The events that followed were a blur. I was taken to the radiology suite, and the ultrasound technician confirmed that my daughter had died. I was admitted to L&D and went from being the on-call physician to being a patient. My obstetrician was on medical leave, so one of my partners became my physician. I chose to be induced rather than wait for spontaneous labor as all I could focus on was getting home to be with my family. My parents had just arrived to celebrate my father's birthday and were staying with us over Christmas.

In parallel with losing my daughter, one of my patients experienced a bilateral femoral neuropathy following a hysterectomy I performed a few days before learning of my unborn daughter's death. She was transferred to a rehabilitation hospital, and I couldn't participate in her care. Not only was I reeling from my own loss, but I did not have privileges at that facility.

It remains the saddest Christmas of my life.

Losing a baby is painfully difficult. Losing a baby while practicing obstetrics is devastating.

If a patient of mine suffers this kind of loss, I usually recommend three weeks off for physical and emotional recovery. After delivering my fourth daughter a few days before Christmas, I planned to do the same. But near the end of the third week, I was terrified of returning to work. I didn't feel psychologically ready to treat patients, so I stayed home for an additional three weeks.

Once I was back at work, I found it emotionally taxing to care for my obstetrical patients. Especially those who shared my due date, women whose bellies were growing when mine was now flat. Because of the special connection we had from being pregnant together, I received lots of questions about what happened and genuine sympathy. That human touch from my patients helped with my healing.

My first night back on call was at the centralized hospital where I had delivered my stillborn daughter. One of the women I was caring for that night had been diagnosed with a fetal demise at twenty-eight weeks, and I would be the physician responsible for her delivery. I honestly felt I wasn't strong enough to be her obstetrician and not let my own tragic experience cloud my judgment. I decided to sit with her and share my sorrow and let her express her grief. We bonded as two women who shared a horrific agony, and it transcended the usual doctor-patient relationship. After that, I felt empowered to continue practicing, knowing I could not only heal but that my experience could help others do the same.

Despite feeling ready to work again at the position I truly thought was my forever job, the part-time, three days per week schedule morphed into at least forty hours plus the in-house night calls at the hospital. My mindset had changed, and I felt it was important to prioritize my needs. I decided to hire an additional nanny to help with the girls, given that I could be gone for twelve hours at a time. Sarah's preschool teacher, Mandy, was looking for an extra job, so she began working as my afternoon nanny. Betsy arrived in the mornings to help the kids with breakfast and take them to school, and Mandy would bring Sarah home from preschool and relieve Betsy, taking care of the children until I returned.

Having two nannies was expensive but worth it as I was able to finish my charting after seeing the last patient at the office while Mandy started the afternoon and early evening routine with the girls.

I'll never forget one of the first days I came home from work after Mandy began helping me. The television wasn't on, and classical music was playing through the stereo speakers. The girls were happily engaged in creating Easter baskets from brown paper garbage sacks. They looked up at me and exclaimed, "Hi, Mommy!" with smiles on their faces. Everyone was happy. The mood was peaceful, not chaotic. Instantly, I felt calmer and knew that I could focus on my career on the days that I was working because the girls were well cared for. This lessened my feelings of unnecessary guilt, which so many working mothers experience.

One Thursday afternoon, my parents were arriving from Austin for the weekend. I was trying to finish a long day of seeing patients, reviewing lab results, and completing notes in the charts after the last patient left at 5:00 pm. In an attempt to be home earlier each day, I had asked my employer to allow me to end my clinic day at 3:00 pm so that I could be with my daughters for what I called "crunch time," which revolved around picking them up from school, helping them with their homework and shuttling them to their various activities. Even though Mandy was caring for my daughters in the afternoons, it was important to *me* to be home between the end of the school day and dinner time. In exchange for being able to leave at 3:00 pm, I offered to see patients during the scheduled lunch break. Sadly, this request was denied as late afternoon appointments were often requested by students and teachers in the community where I practiced.

On the day my parents arrived for the weekend, I wasn't there to greet them. Thankfully, I had prepared our home for their visit with all the grocery shopping done, fresh flowers in vases, the guest room freshened, and menus planned to include cocktail hour.

I had made all these preparations and wasn't able to be there.

I was trapped behind a stack of charts with seemingly hours of more work left to do, and I began to feel tears welling up in my eyes. Despite my very best efforts at balancing my career with family life, I felt like such a failure, just as I had with my first job at the cancer center. Here I was, working late while everyone at home was starting the weekend.

I had had enough and hastily wrote out a resignation letter on a piece of notebook paper giving thirty days' notice.

I left my dark office and drove home… and began planning what would be my second leave from clinical practice.

* * *

THE GIRLS WERE NOW TWO, four, and six, and attending three different schools with three different drop off and pick up times. At the start of my second leave, my plan was to stop working completely until Maggie entered kindergarten, which was three years away. This would be a true sabbatical.

My days were filled with being home in the mornings, feeding the girls breakfast, taking them to school (while wearing my workout clothes instead of scrubs), exercising with friends, running errands, enjoying hobbies, and sleeping in my own bed every night without the underlying anxiety of possibly being called in to the hospital.

I was in heaven.

I felt like a "real mom" and savored the relationships I was building with my new "mommy friends," many of whom had given up their careers to stay home with their children. I began volunteering at the girls' schools, participating in carpools, and having playgroup parties at my house. My sister Sam, whose son John was two years younger than Maggie, lived only ten minutes away. She had decided to stay home after her boy was born, and we spent a lot of time together. I immersed myself in the joy of unstructured time watching our children play together while we chatted and cooked and solved the world's problems.

This was bliss. I felt like I was being the "mommy" that my mom had been to me and my siblings.

I didn't miss working at all.

Then, only eight months into my second leave, the phone rang while I was supervising a rambunctious group of preschoolers in our swimming pool. The call was from my most recent employer, who inquired if I might be interested in covering for one of the physicians who was out on medical leave. Coincidentally, the physician I would be covering for was the obstetrician who took care of me when I delivered my fourth daughter.

I pondered the request and let the caller know that my daughters' drop-off and pick-up times were at three different schools, and it was important that I was home with them in the afternoons. Therefore, I could only be available on Monday, Wednesday, and Friday from 9:00 am to 1:00 pm. I would also not be able to help with in-house L&D call but offered to assist in the operating room if the commute wasn't more than thirty minutes each way. I added that I would need help with medmal insurance as I no longer maintained coverage and expected an hourly rate of compensation for my time.

I fully expected a polite refusal, yet my requests were accepted, followed by a plea to begin working in four days.

And thus, my second leave abruptly ended.

Two and a half years ahead of schedule.

- *Juggling the obligations of a demanding career with caring for children is stressful but can be alleviated by learning to rely on the help of others as well as delegating responsibilities.*

- *It is important to set expectations with your employer that there will be times when taking time off to care for your family will be necessary.*

INTRODUCTION TO LOCUM TENENS

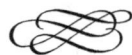

$\mathcal{M}$y second leave ended in early 1998, before the use of the Internet was standard operating procedure. My former employer sent a batch of re-hire paperwork via courier to my home with instructions to fill it out and call them when it was completed. I promptly finished it, and a second courier picked it up.

Working on Fridays was going to be a challenge because it was Betsy's day off, and I didn't have any childcare. I was nervous about being able to get the girls dropped off at their three different schools, drive thirty minutes to downtown Houston, and secure a spot in the parking garage in time for the first patient scheduled at 9:00 am.

I enlisted the help of one of my new mommy friends, Ami, and asked if I dropped Sarah off at her house in the morning, would she please take her to school so that I could get to work on time? Ami was more than happy to do this as our kids were classmates, and they could play together while she helped her younger son get ready for the day.

It was a win-win.

And off I went to downtown Houston, in December, eight months after my plan to not work again until Maggie was in kindergarten.

Business attire: Check. Briefcase: Check.

I was both nervous and giddy with excitement regarding this unexpected career opportunity.

I entered downtown marveling at the Christmas decorations, parked in the garage, and ascended the escalator inside a tall office building lined floor to ceiling with windows, which were bordered by twinkling holiday lights. I thought I had died and gone to heaven and was living inside a movie script set in New York City.

Was this really happening?

I arrived at the clinic where I was scheduled to see patients for the physician who was on medical leave and was greeted by smiling front desk staff and nurses who told me how much they appreciated my help as they escorted me to my pod.

For the next four hours, I rifled through charts, introduced myself to patients as the "substitute doctor," and practiced my craft. Women streamed in and out of the office with Ob/Gyn concerns that I was able to take care of much more easily than I had anticipated.

Everyone was happy.

The patients were happy because there was a physician in the office to care for them. The nurses and staff were happy because phone call messages, prescription refill requests, and lab results were addressed in a timely manner. The physician who was out on medical leave was happy because her practice was left in good hands, allowing her to properly recover from her accident.

I was happy because this position gave me the chance to maintain my Ob/Gyn skill set while earning income on a part-time basis.

Through word of mouth, this would be the first of several assignments I took following the end of my second leave from clinical practice. My requests were the same with each: Monday, Wednesday, and Friday from 9:00 am to 1:00 pm, an hourly rate of pay, no call, and coverage for malpractice insurance.

My daughters never knew I was at work.

I was pleased with my newfound "method" of being able to take care of family obligations while practicing as an Ob/Gyn. The blend of sporadic part-time local locum tenens opportunities was a dream come true. I was very involved with my girls' schools, extracurricular activities, and community commitments, and I enjoyed the camaraderie of other moms in our neighborhood.

- *When negotiating, establish your boundaries and stick to them.*
- *Don't be tempted to plunge in with both feet when starting a new venture. Test the waters first.*

FIRST EXPERIENCE WITH
PRIVATE PRACTICE

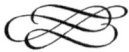

*O*ne day, a former colleague from residency, Dr. Peters, called me out of the blue regarding a job opportunity. I had approached him a year or so earlier about coming to help with his practice. At that time, he felt I was "too expensive" to hire.

This time, his wife, who was also an Ob/Gyn, was pregnant with their third child. She wanted to take a year off from practicing medicine to stay home with their three sons.

My colleague asked if I would be willing to take care of his wife's patients while she was out.

I honestly wasn't ready to work more than the twelve hours per week I was currently committed to, and was initially hesitant to even consider this job.

I asked Dr. Peters for a part-time option with minimal to no night call, and we negotiated for sixteen hours per week. This worked out to be four half days each week with a few night calls per month. He offered me a salary rather than per diem pay as I had received for previous locums, plus medmal coverage. Additionally, I would learn the basics of running a private practice, which was a new skill set for me. It seemed like an excellent opportunity, so I agreed to the terms.

So here I was, less than two years into my locum tenens work, when I plunged into new long-term employment, this time with colleagues I had worked with during residency. The office was ten minutes from home and ten minutes from each of the girls' schools. The only concerning issue was that the hospitals where our group did deliveries, made rounds, and performed surgeries would be a forty-minute commute for me. Thankfully, the other members of our group lived closer to the hospitals than I did and could cover for me when necessary.

The demographics of the patient population we served demanded that I work one of those half days in the afternoon. This conflicted with my daughters' after-school schedules as well as when Betsy needed to leave for the day. My solution was to have Betsy drop the girls off at my office on the days I saw patients in the afternoon. The girls enjoyed coming to the clinic where they could get a snack from the pharmacy in our building and work quietly on their homework at my big desk. Wild peacocks often roamed in the parking lot, which added to the girls' excitement.

After the first year, Dr. Peter's wife returned to the office, and my salary arrangement changed. She saw patients on one of the days I wasn't there, and we set up a job-sharing schedule that allowed us to see our own patients.

I was introduced to a business term called "cost center," where my income would be based on the revenue I generated from patient care minus my portion of the overhead expenses. It was the first time in my career that I worked within an "eat what you kill" business model that incentivizes physicians to increase the volume of patients seen in the office and the number of procedures performed at the hospital to generate more revenue.

I began to learn more about the basics of running a private medical practice. The joint expenses of rent, utilities, payroll, and supplies were shared on a prorated basis among the members of the group, but other expenses such as medmal insurance were not. It was 2001, prior to the tort reform in Texas, and Ob/Gyns in Harris County paid one of the highest medical liability insurance premium rates in the US.

I learned that reimbursement from health insurance companies to physicians was highly variable. The amount paid for an office visit or procedure was less than the amount billed, varied by payor, and was not received in a timely manner relative to the date of service. For obstetric patients, payment for prenatal, delivery, and postpartum care sometimes didn't occur until after the baby was born and the mom had completed her postpartum visit six weeks later. Because of these inconsistencies, it was difficult to predict the amount of revenue earned each month despite the business expenses staying the same.

I became disheartened. My income during the second year with this group dropped by fifty percent when compared to the salary I earned the first year, even though I saw the same volume of patients and did the same number of procedures.

There were, however, positive aspects to this job.

I enjoyed taking care of my own patients and bonding with them and I enjoyed learning the business side of medicine. Most importantly, I was still able to work part-time and maintain the work-life balance my family was accustomed to.

But over time, I found that balancing my commitments to patients with obligations to my family became increasingly difficult. This was primarily due to after-hours call responsibilities and completion of administrative tasks such as following up on lab and imaging results, prescription refill requests, and answering messages from nurses.

These were the same issues I had experienced at my second job with the multispecialty group, which led to my abrupt resignation!

Once again, I felt that I had failed as a physician and was inadequate in taking care of my children. I began to seriously question my decision to leave sporadic local locum tenens work for private practice.

Despite living forty-five minutes from the hospital, I tried to deliver all my own patients, even when I wasn't on call. I felt a special connection to each unborn baby as if she were my child.

I only missed deliveries when I was on vacation, except for one pivotal instance.

Sarah participated in year-round soccer, and one afternoon, I was on my way to drop her off at practice with the plan to deliver one of my pregnant patients later that evening.

However, my patient went into labor at the time I dropped Sarah off, and the forty-five-minute commute to the hospital significantly lengthened during the Houston rush hour.

Suddenly, an L&D nurse called me to let me know my patient was progressing rapidly and would be ready for delivery soon.

It was one of the first times in my Ob/Gyn career that I felt I wouldn't be able to make it to the hospital in time for a delivery. I faced the dilemma of trying to navigate very heavy traffic to get to the hospital with the option of asking one of my practice partners to step in for me. I also felt guilty for even considering going to the hospital, given that this would require a complete restructuring of the afternoon and evening plans I had made for my daughters.

I decided to contact one of my practice partners and asked if she could cover for me. My partner was not on call, and my request meant that she also had to revise her afternoon and evening plans.

This was a defining moment in my career. I decided I probably shouldn't practice obstetrics anymore due to the unpredictability of caring for maternity patients.

Looking back, I realize this conflict wasn't the end of the world. My patient had an uncomplicated delivery of a healthy baby and did well. My practice partner understood the dilemma I was facing and was more than happy to step in. I imagine that my girls didn't realize what I was feeling, and their afternoon and evening went on as usual.

A hack I learned from this and other experiences I faced when juggling after-hours patient care with family commitments is to always have a backup plan.

DISGRUNTLED staff began to complain about the girls coming to the office for a few hours on Wednesday afternoons as they weren't allowed to do the same for their children. I was disappointed, as the girls' presence wasn't disruptive, and this enabled me to be a more productive physician by seeing patients during a time frame that was in high demand. But the practice administrator requested that the girls no longer come to the office.

The lengthy commute back and forth from the hospitals for rounds, deliveries, and surgeries worsened. Since I was the only member of our group that lived so far from the hospitals, I asked my partners if I could obtain privileges at a hospital closer to home while remaining part of the main call group. Due to my childcare issues, I no longer wanted to see patients in the afternoons and asked if I could work through lunch instead.

I was determined to negotiate a solution and drew up a mini business plan with an updated office and call schedule and felt confident that it would be approved.

It wasn't, and my increasing frustrations with the company's policies led me to begin seeking opportunities that wouldn't require obstetrics.

- *Utilize your network of friends, family members, and childcare providers to pitch in when you need them and offer to reciprocate when you can.*
- *Take the time to learn the basics of running a private medical practice.*

NEXT PIVOT—RETURN TO ACADEMIA

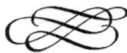

*I*n my heart, I knew that the current private practice situation would not be feasible long term. The girls were getting busier. Jane was in middle school, and during my nightly walks with my best friend, I continually complained about the stresses associated with the job.

I decided to contact one of the nurse practitioners I had worked with at the cancer center to see if she knew of any opportunities for a gynecology position. The postings on the job boards all required Ob, and practicing obstetrics was no longer conducive to the work-life balance I desired.

My colleague let me know that my former position had recently been posted. However, it was now a full-time faculty appointment requiring at least forty hours per week.

At this point in my career, my "mommy network" was robust, and Jane was just a few years away from driving. I felt that with well-organized planning and coordinating care for the girls in the afternoons, I could commit to a full-time position. Especially if it wouldn't require obstetrics.

The salary was almost five-fold more than I was earning by working part-time as a private practice Ob/Gyn. Additionally, the benefits were enticing. They matched retirement contributions, provided medmal coverage, disability coverage, life insurance, paid time off, a CME stipend, and promised an annual bonus. Plus, I would have the opportunity to work in academic medicine again with some of the best and brightest physicians I'd ever known.

At dinner that night, I brought up the opportunity, and my daughters' eyes twinkled with excitement. I could feel their support. This was important to me as I weighed the decision of whether to go full-time again after working shorter weeks for ten years.

I accepted the offer and jumped right in with both feet.

Returning to the cancer center was exhilarating. I enjoyed working with renowned physicians, curating a niche practice, collaborating on research projects, participating on institutional committees, writing scientific articles, performing complex gynecologic surgeries, traveling to give presentations, and teaching nurse practitioners, residents, and fellows. I found that contributing to the care of oncology patients was unexpectedly rewarding and professionally fulfilling.

In contrast to the excitement of returning to academia, my marriage to my daughters' father became increasingly strained. We were both working full-time as physicians and I was climbing the academic ladder of success. His mother was ill with metastatic cancer and received her treatments in Houston, staying with us every few weeks. I felt as though I was doing most of the caregiving while he worked harder and wasn't home much. We drifted apart and despite seeking counseling, our marriage sadly ended.

Over the next few years, I was thrust into juggling the care of my teenage daughters and our family home with my career obligations as a single mother. At work, things also took a turn. Although I had been looking forward to being promoted to professor, which came with a significant salary increase and benefits, my department chair retired, and a new chairman was appointed.

And the culture in the department began to change.

I was no longer involved in important decisions.

In a meeting with the vice-chairman of the department and my section chief, I was given a negative critique of my professional performance and placed on probation. I felt their concerns were unfounded and set out to prove them wrong.

I earnestly began fulfilling the responsibilities the vice-chairman and section chief had told me I was deficient in. Creating agendas, attending more required meetings, being more punctual and communicative with staff.

When the time for my annual review arrived, I was looking forward to being told that my probation had ended and that I would receive my promotion.

I walked into the chairman's office, and my section chief was present. She had never come to these meetings before. Things didn't feel right.

Neither of them had smiles on their faces. The corner office, which usually glimmered with positivity as sunlight streamed through floor-to-ceiling windows, felt cloudy.

The mood was foreboding.

I was handed a paper that indicated my contract was not being renewed at the end of the calendar year, giving me four months' notice.

I was shocked and exclaimed, "I'm on track to be promoted to full professor in a few weeks. I've done everything I was asked to do. I'm a single mom with three teenage daughters!"

Silence in the room.

I pushed the paper back across the desk, unsigned.

"I resign," I said. "My last day will be in three weeks."

Then, I walked out.

I met Wilson shortly after my separation from the girls' father and he was incredibly supportive during the events that led to the unfortunate end of my academic career. I had begun exploring job opportunities closer to where he lived in the event I decided to move.

I knew I could start over again. But I never expected I'd *have* to leave.

NEW LIFE DIRECTION

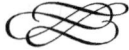

*D*espite the circumstances, leaving my nine-year academic position was difficult.

I felt like a professional failure.

Wilson steadied me, grounded me, and helped me feel sane. We began planning a future together in parallel with my exhaustive search for jobs, but positions for an Ob/Gyn who hadn't practiced obstetrics in over ten years were almost unheard of.

During my tenure at the cancer center, part of my clinical responsibilities included working at the county hospital. One of my medical school classmates, Mary, was also working there and we renewed our friendship after having not seen each other since graduation, over twenty years earlier.

Mary is a renowned academician and mentor. She invited me to join a group of women colleagues with whom she socialized regularly. We used to meet at fine restaurants and wine bars to discuss our careers and personal lives and support each other during times of transition. The laughter and incredible conversations transported me to a world outside of medicine where I could feel human and connected to other professional women.

When my contract wasn't renewed at the cancer center, Mary and

I bonded even more closely, as she had also been through an eerily similar experience.

Mary connected me with a colleague working close to the area I would be moving to, and this physician knew of two gynecologists looking for a partner. I immediately pursued this as I felt it would be my only chance to continue working without practicing obstetrics.

THIS GYNECOLOGY-ONLY OPPORTUNITY was a true private practice with no financial or credentialing support from a corporation or hospital system. I had briefly experienced the "eat what you kill" business model before during the last years of my part-time Ob/Gyn private practice. Because of this, I felt I possessed the basic fund of knowledge regarding what to expect in terms of running a medical business.

Despite my excitement regarding this new venture, deep down, I was petrified.

I realized there was a major drawback to this position, as very few of my patients from the cancer center would follow me, given that most of them lived out of town. I would need to build the business from the ground up, which meant learning how to market my services to prospective new patients.

Still, I continued to explore the opportunity by meeting with the senior physician of the group who had recently dropped obstetrics. She had a good reputation and patient following in the area. We seemed aligned in our philosophies and approaches to patient care. And we both loved to operate.

I also met with the office manager who helped me with credentialing for insurance plans, which I knew nothing about and had never needed to do before. She suggested marketing ideas, about which I was also naïve; all my previous employers had done the marketing for me.

I toured the office and expressed to the team that I planned to take a few months off between jobs so that I could get my bearings on exiting the academic position and spend as much time with Maggie as possible before she went away to college.

I had savings to support myself, but I was overwhelmed with everything that was happening: Leaving my job at the cancer center, planning a wedding, starting a new practice, getting my house ready to sell, and becoming an empty nester.

I just needed to breathe.

Despite my plans to take a few months off, the senior partner and office manager urged me to start earlier than my projected timeline so that I could help with the shared overhead expenses.

Reluctantly, I agreed, and the week after I officially left the cancer center, I began working in a new private practice with two other physicians whom I barely knew.

I truly did not know what I was doing and felt like I had been thrown into a swimming pool without knowing how to swim.

I worked diligently to attract new patients by networking with local physicians, joining the Chamber of Commerce, placing low-cost advertisements in community newsletters, printing business cards, and developing a simple website. It didn't take long before I began to enjoy my new gynecology private practice, sharing office space and overhead expenses with two other mid-career women Ob/Gyns. The clinic was designed for two physicians, but we made it work by creating a schedule where only two of us were in at the same time. There were only two official physicians' offices, so I converted a storage closet into my workspace.

I was motivated by my determination to succeed as well as the fear of financial insecurity.

My schedule consisted of seeing patients two and a half days a week and performing major gynecologic surgeries at the hospital once a week. We had a surgery day in our office once a month on a Friday for minor gynecologic surgeries, which included endometrial ablations, hysteroscopies, and loop electrosurgical excision procedures (LEEPs). An anesthesia group would come to our suite accompanied by ancillary surgical staff who would bring the necessary supplies and equipment. These procedures were performed under intravenous (IV) sedation with airway management. I learned that the reimbursements from insurance companies were much higher for doing these procedures in a clinic setting rather than in the operating room at the hospital.

Despite the seemingly smooth operation of day surgery and seductively higher insurance compensation, I wasn't completely comfortable with this concept given that our suite was on the fifth floor of a free-standing medical professional building without direct access to the hospital in the event of a complication. But with time, my fears were alleviated as our patients did well and were appreciative of not having to go to the hospital for their surgeries, as well as the calmer environment we created for them. As surgeons, we were able to perform many more procedures in a day than when done at the surgery center due to a quicker turnover time between cases.

Our camaraderie as a threesome grew, and so did the volume of new patients booking appointments with me.

We shared night and weekend call with another group of gynecology-only physicians in our area. This group also performed office surgeries on Fridays, so weekend calls primarily consisted of minor issues that these post-operative patients were experiencing.

I learned Excel so that I could create spreadsheets that tracked each business expense and bank deposit as well as the number of patients seen and surgeries performed. My income goal was lofty yet still below what I had earned at the cancer center and based on what I needed to afford my living expenses. I no longer had benefits, so I purchased a COBRA policy for health insurance along with disability coverage.

But the revenue coming in minus the overhead expenses was significantly less than what I had hoped for. My savings wouldn't last long, and I realized that I needed to explore additional income streams.

At the time, there were minimal resources available to help physicians explore other sources of revenue. Moonlighting options were limited to working shifts in urgent care settings, which I wasn't eligible to do without the required training in emergency medicine or primary care.

I began connecting with recruiters regarding Ob/Gyn locum

tenens positions as well as searching job boards for both clinical and non-clinical jobs. Mary, whose connections had led to my current private practice situation, was also in pursuit of side gigs. She became a champion for my success by sending me information regarding any prospect that came her way that she thought might be a good fit for me.

But almost all locum tenens opportunities for an Ob/Gyn centered on practicing obstetrics. That was what was in demand owing to the increasing physician shortage, especially in rural areas.

I narrowed my search to the scant opportunities available for strictly Gyn positions. My experiences with local locum tenens assignments during my second leave from practice came in handy because they taught me about the art of negotiating. It was important that the side gigs not interfere with my clinic schedule, so I was clear with the recruiting companies about what I would be willing to offer.

Ultimately, I found work as a per diem physician for two local clinics on days I wasn't scheduled to see patients in my office or operate. One of these opportunities was working for a state-funded clinic that provided care to patients who were underinsured. My responsibilities were limited to office gynecology, and I was paid an hourly rate. It was a challenging position given the limited resources available to patients who needed consultative care beyond what could be provided in the clinical setting. Most of the patients were non-English speaking, and without a readily available translation service, I fumbled with my limited medical Spanish. I relied on the bilingual nurses to help me.

The job at the state-funded clinic lasted only a few months, but I was able to find another opening shortly thereafter at another state facility for underserved patients. This clinic was established through a partnership with one of the medical schools in Houston. My responsibilities included providing prenatal care as well as routine gynecological care. This experience helped me begin to relearn obstetrics in the outpatient setting, which became crucial to eventually being able to work full scope Ob/Gyn locums.

Through these two clinic experiences, I felt hopeful about my ability to balance the demands of my growing private practice with working another job to make ends meet.

I determinedly continued to pursue Ob/Gyn locum tenens work. But despite the growing shortage in the specialty and my eagerness to work, I received rejection after rejection due to my lack of recent hospital obstetrical experience.

I was beyond frustrated!

A ray of hope surfaced when I learned of a formal re-training program for physicians who have stepped away from practicing or who have decided to drop obstetrics. Very few formal re-training programs exist, and this one just happened to be nearby.

I excitedly applied, was accepted, and eagerly awaited the start of this two-year program. I had devised a schedule where I would be able to continue seeing patients two and a half days a week in my practice, operate, and complete the requirements for the program on the weekends.

A few weeks before the program was set to start, I was informed that it had folded. I would be first on the acceptance list if the program reopened.

Another stumbling block.

Now what?

- *Tap into the professional connections you've made when searching for new opportunities*
- *When pivoting to a new job, be transparent with your patients so that they may continue to see you if they are able*
- *Utilize the resources provided by your state medical board when starting a new practice*

LEARNING MORE ABOUT THE
BUSINESS SIDE OF MEDICINE

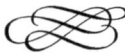

S ince I knew how to run a lemonade stand, balance my checkbook, and create homegrown Excel spreadsheets for my private practice, I foolishly assumed I understood the basics of running a business. It was a simple math problem, really. Revenue minus overhead expenses equals income. But terms like accounts payable, accounts receivable, and financial forecasting seemed more abstract. I felt that by learning additional business skills, I could optimize my practice finances. I also thought that earning an advanced business degree might lead to possible hospital administration positions in the future.

But the notion of studying for yet another entrance exam and taking college course prerequisites at this phase of my career was intimidating, so I temporarily abandoned this dream.

One day, a brochure arrived in the mail for a hybrid business program for healthcare professionals at an Ivy League school in New England. My eyes glazed with excitement as I discussed the option with my husband. There would be four on-site sessions lasting anywhere from five days to two weeks over a one-and-a-half-year timeframe. When not in residence, the program required twenty hours per week devoted to remote learning, which consisted of reading, online lectures, and individual and group projects. The class size would be limited.

With Wilson's encouragement, I applied.

I was enjoying lunch with my friend Mary when my cell phone rang, and the caller ID displayed the name of the admissions office. I ignored it partly to not appear rude, but even more because I was afraid it might be yet another rejection.

Mary encouraged me to call them back immediately, which I did as I was driving home. The news was positive. I had been accepted into the program.

Now I just had to figure out how I was going to afford it.

I learned from my accountant that earnings from my practice could pay for educational expenses for its employees. I was an employee of my business, so I was able to pay my tuition for the program with practice earnings. Additionally, the travel and lodging expenses incurred during my residential sessions would be eligible for reimbursement through my practice.

And the autonomy of being in private practice meant I could travel whenever I wanted to.

I loved going back to school, out of state, in a learning environment that was completely different from my experiences as an undergraduate and medical student. There were about forty-five people in my class from all over the country, half of whom were physicians. The remainder of my classmates were hospital administrators, attorneys, policymakers, nurses, healthcare business owners, and insurance executives.

The first two-week session necessitated living in the dorm on campus. We were transported back in time to our years in college, leading to somewhat sophomoric behavior. It didn't take long for our class to bond as we spent late nights studying and visiting the local bars and restaurants.

It was exhilarating to be learning side-by-side with such a diverse group of mid-career health professionals. I thrived in this environment and looked forward to the remote sessions when I got back home.

In parallel with returning to school, I continued to pursue side gig opportunities to meet my financial goals, but I received a constant cascade of rejections from recruiting firms due to my gap in practicing obstetrics in the hospital setting.

One of my classmates in the program was a family medicine physician with Ob training who was from rural Kansas. The town in which Dr. Arbus practiced had a population of only 2,000 people, yet they were delivering thirty babies a month at the Critical Access Hospital (CAH), where he also held the position of chief medical officer (CMO). This was a remarkable volume for a small rural hospital. What was also impressive was that comprehensive Ob/Gyn care was provided to patients by a group of family medicine physicians who were cross-trained in women's health.

I told Dr. Arbus about my private practice situation and desire to increase my income, as well as my lack of recent work in obstetrics. He devised a plan where I could travel to Kansas to help teach gynecologic surgery to family medicine residents rotating through the CAH who did not receive sufficient training in this area. In exchange, I would re-train in obstetrics by working in parallel with the family medicine physicians on staff. The plan was to travel to Kansas once a month, see patients in the clinic, operate, teach, and take night call.

Our entrepreneurial idea was supported by Dr. Arbus's chief executive officer (CEO), a non-physician, who had also completed the same business school program a year ahead of our class. I flew out to this area in remote Kansas for an interview and tour.

Everything was set after the interview. Using my experience during my second leave from practice when I negotiated the terms of local locum tenens agreements, I was able to negotiate a per diem rate of pay. The next steps were signing a contract, obtaining a Kansas medical license, and proposing some work dates.

As I was eagerly waiting to travel to Kansas for my first shift, I encountered a significant stumbling block.

How would my Kansas liability coverage be paid?

The hospital administrators in Kansas felt they couldn't assume this cost and given that there was no way for me to afford Ob/Gyn medmal out of state, the negotiations halted.

Unfortunately, this would become a recurrent issue for future opportunities given the high cost of malpractice insurance for obstetrics. In Texas, I only maintained coverage for gynecology.

Naturally, I was dejected as I felt this opportunity would check a lot of boxes. I would have re-learned obstetrical skills, been able to teach again, supplemented my private practice income, and been able to travel to a remote rural area to serve a patient population with gaps in care.

But despite my disappointment, I realized that I could now realistically explore opportunities for locum tenens jobs outside the state of Texas *if* the employer agreed to cover the cost of medmal insurance.

This was huge.

And thus, the pursuit of locum tenens jobs in other states began.

- *It is not necessary to get an advanced business degree to learn how to run a medical practice*
- *Understanding the viewpoint of all stakeholders is important when negotiating an agreement*
- *Never stop learning*
- *Don't abandon hope when your situation seems desperate*
- *What seems like an insurmountable setback can be a stepping stone to something better*
- *Through perseverance, your path can be refined, and you can thrive*

HOW I CREATED A MICRO PRACTICE

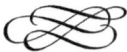

*T*he three of us who shared overhead expenses began to grow apart. Our business philosophies diverged with my senior partner's desire to focus on aesthetic gynecology and my other partner's initiation of online supplement sales through a multilevel marketing strategy. I felt these tactics were not evidence-based and didn't align with my core values. One of the partners left the group and a chiropractor and his wife began subleasing space from us, which made the office crowded. We were three independent practices with significantly different styles sharing employees and office space. It became necessary to consider the possibility of going completely solo.

While on a weekend reunion retreat with some of my business school colleagues, I was lamenting the inadequate insurance reimbursements, divergence from my partners, and my frustration with not being able to earn a decent living after three years in private practice.

One of my former classmates, Dr. Evan, suggested that I consider starting a micro practice. I had never heard of this term, but with his encouragement, I began reading everything I could on the subject.

In simple terms, a micro practice is exactly that. Small.

Small in scope. Small in overhead. Small in number of employees. Small in office square footage.

The key is to operate the business as leanly as possible with few employees, no partners, and minimum exam rooms. This not only maximizes income for the solo practitioner but also allows for optimal professional autonomy when designing the office flow, training staff, controlling the number of patients seen, and determining which types of appointments are given at what times. I planned to continue offering the same services as I had been except for on-site surgeries. Instead, these minor gynecologic procedures would be done in the ambulatory surgery center (ASC).

My micro practice would be a true solo endeavor.

During my residency, I vividly remember visiting my dentist and being impressed with the warmth and hominess of the office environment. It was located inside a small house that had been remodeled into a dental office. The décor was just as one would expect inside a well-kept home, very unlike the typical sterile environment of a medical practice. There were little touches here and there that infused an atmosphere of relaxation and personalized care.

At the time, I thought to myself, "Someday I hope to have an office like this. Why not deliver gynecologic care to patients in a setting that exudes warmth and calmness while lessening anxiety?"

With my professional divorce behind me, I was ready, excited, and nervous to finally have the opportunity to implement this idea by opening a new solo micro practice.

I successfully recruited two of the medical assistants I had been working with to come with me. Dee would become my office manager and work in the front; Christina would become my patient care coordinator and work in the back.

Both Dee and Christina were as excited as I was regarding this new venture, and we worked as a team to launch it.

There were so many details to take care of, including finding a new office space, notifying patients, integrating a new electronic health record (EHR) and billing service, stocking supplies and appropriate equipment, and organizing a move.

The memories of writing out a list during my first leave from practice of what I would need to open a gynecology office came flooding back.

My office manager, Dee, was unmatched in her dedication and work ethic and was devoted to my mission and plan. She orchestrated so much of the logistics of what needed to be done. We brainstormed my exit strategy, and she was invaluable in guiding me through this process.

My last day at the former office was in late December, and we started seeing patients in the new location in early January.

When I shared overhead expenses with the other physicians, we joined a management services organization (MSO) to help gain higher rates of reimbursement from health insurance companies. Although we did receive increased amounts from payors, I felt that the fees I was paying to the MSO weren't worth it. One of the first changes I made upon going solo was to dissolve this business relationship.

The dissolution of the partnership with the MSO was trickier than I had anticipated. All the payor contracts were between the MSO using its National Provider Identifier (NPI) number and the insurance companies. Therefore, I had to renegotiate and set up new contracts with insurance companies using my individual NPI number. This took several months. Additionally, the transfer of patient information from the existing EHR into the new one did not go smoothly, even though the electronic health records vendor was the same. The customization of the platform for the MSO was proprietary, so all my patients' information and files had to be purchased and downloaded onto a hard drive. I then had to renegotiate a new contract with the *same* EHR vendor to use the *same* platform at a higher cost than what I had been paying through the MSO.

I learned the difficult lesson that solo practitioners don't have much power when negotiating for services from merchants when compared to large group practices, and this didn't just apply to health insurance contracts.

Dee & Christina painstakingly printed each patient's record from the old program, then scanned it into the new software at the time of the patient's initial visit to our new clinic. Countless tedious hours were spent transferring patient records between essentially the same EHRs.

Another exhausting and frustrating step in moving forward.

Dee was indispensable in helping me re-credential as an independent physician with all the payor contracts. Although she had never worked in this role before, her years of working alongside office managers in several Ob/Gyn practices gave her the necessary skills that she applied to running our practice.

My micro practice is set up as part-time, which helps keep overhead costs low and allows for the following benefits:

1. The ability to negotiate a lower malpractice insurance rate
2. Keep daily patient volume low, allowing more time with each patient
3. Able to adapt scheduling to accommodate other jobs (side gigs)
4. Option to sublease space during days when not in the office
5. Employee satisfaction and retention due to flexibility of work hours
6. The ability to optimize work-life balance with time for self-care, family and friends, hobbies, and traveling

I truly view my micro practice as *our* practice," given that it takes a dedicated team of like-minded individuals, regardless of their responsibilities within the company, to fully care for patients. I had learned management skills in the business school program and knew it was important to communicate regularly with my employees and to expand their responsibilities as much as possible within the scope of their licenses.

From the time an appointment is made until a plan for the patient is implemented, all aspects of each person's care are a joint effort between the three of us.

Practicing as a solo gynecologist in a micro setting has been rewarding.

My patients are happy, I am professionally satisfied, and Dee and Christina, whom I view as my "other" daughters, have the work-life balance they need so they can attend to their families. This is the same arrangement I tried so hard to achieve when my girls were growing up.

With a top-rated EHR, I can access my patients' charts remotely to take care of messages, review lab and imaging results, and authorize prescription refills even when I am not physically present in the office. This functionality became more important as I began working more side gigs, especially those that involved travel.

Because I am completely solo, I take call for my surgical patients by providing them with my cell phone number, which they can call or text for after-hours concerns or emergencies. When traveling out of the forty-eight contiguous states, I share call with another gynecology-only physician nearby who covers for me, and likewise, I cover for her when she travels long distances.

Unfortunately, the setbacks continued.

Shortly after the transition, Hurricane Harvey dumped fifty inches of rain over the area in two days. Roads were impassable, homes were flooded, the power grid was compromised, and schools and businesses were closed. It was a true disaster.

I was unable to see patients in my office or perform surgeries for over two weeks. Even when the power and internet were restored, a significant number of my patients took months to recover from the storm's impact on their jobs, homes, and emotional well-being. Unfortunately, the fallout from this weather catastrophe significantly impacted my practice revenue.

Through it all, Dee, Christina, and I continued to work diligently to maintain a lean business model. But the reality of not sharing overhead with other physicians, coupled with having exited the MSO and receiving lower insurance reimbursements, made me thankful that I had continued the pursuit of side gigs.

I boosted my practice income with the addition of 1099 independent contractor jobs brokered between employers and my business corporation to help pay my overhead expenses. I felt optimistic that I could keep the practice going, take care of my patients, and pay my staff.

- *Discounts for medical liability insurance are available to physicians who are first-time private practice owners*
- *Train your employees to cross cover for each other—this will save payroll costs*
- *Shop for pre-owned office furniture and instruments*

LOCUM TENENS 2.0—WHEN A SIDE GIG BECOMES A MAIN GIG

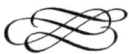

As I previously mentioned, moonlighting opportunities have historically been limited to physicians who can work at free-standing urgent care centers or emergency departments, which is not a scenario typically available to an Ob/Gyn.

Over the past decade, the depth and breadth of secondary jobs, or "side gigs," available to doctors has significantly increased. Both clinical and non-clinical options now exist to earn extra income, which can lead to more financial security and less burnout.

Some of the more common ways a doctor can build a career portfolio include locum tenens, expert witness testimony, telemedicine, medical director positions, utilization review, paid speaking, and medical writing. There are numerous books, podcasts, and social media groups that specifically focus on this strategy, whether it's to pay off student debt, help with practice overhead expenses, defray the cost of children's college education, or buy a new house.

I've been fortunate to have explored several side gig opportunities. Each has its strengths and weaknesses.

Locum tenens is Latin for "to take the place of," and my first experiences with locum tenens jobs following my second leave from practice were positive and influenced by what I had observed my mother do during her "second career."

When my four siblings and I were young, Mom put her career on hold and worked part-time as a school crossing guard for the elementary school on our street. She knew all the children in our neighborhood. Once it was time for my parents to plan financially for the five of us to go to college, my mother went back to work. Over the next twenty years, she sequentially managed several real estate offices and ultimately a pediatrician's office, where our family doctor shared his practice with two other physicians. Mom's forte was reorganization and being able to rapidly assimilate into a new work environment, implementing positive changes while maintaining the existing company culture.

Inspired by and encouraged by my mom, that's how I view my work as a locum tenens physician. Traveling to different hospitals in different states and quickly adapting to a new work environment. Each assignment is like starting over again. I'm required to learn a different EHR system, new hospital policies and procedures, and adjust to the regional customs and climate, all while taking care of patients with respect for the existing culture.

Although the opportunity in Kansas through my business school classmate fell through when they could not subsidize my medmal insurance, that experience encouraged me to look outside the state for locum tenens work.

I cast my net beyond Texas by connecting with multiple recruiting companies that I found online. In the beginning, I would answer every text, phone call, and email from the recruiters in hopes of securing work. As I had done before, I established clear boundaries regarding when I would be available for shifts as well as how far I was willing to travel.

My stipulations were that I could only work a long weekend shift, arriving on a Thursday evening and leaving on a Sunday afternoon so as not to interfere with my micro practice schedule.

Despite multiple conversations with recruiters, during some of which I literally begged for work, I continued to receive rejections due to my lack of recent obstetrical experience.

I would arduously try to persuade the recruiters to consider my candidacy given my skill set in advanced laparoscopic surgery combined with my experience working at the state-funded prenatal clinic for underserved patients.

"I can perform advanced laparoscopic surgery; therefore, I am confident I can perform an emergency C-section!" I would exclaim.

But two main issues kept surfacing. The lack of having performed fifty deliveries within the past two years coupled with the cost of malpractice insurance. On several occasions, I offered to work for half the daily rate and shadow another physician until I reached the obligatory delivery requirement, a number set by the recruiting companies. As a locum tenens, liability insurance is paid for by the recruiting agency; therefore, they are assuming risk when you contract with them to work. When I discovered this, I offered to pay for my own medmal policy. This idea was also rejected.

There was no way I could get hired without performing the requisite number of deliveries. And there seemed to be no way to achieve that goal.

I was financially stressed and had been given a glimmer of hope with the Kansas experience, so I didn't give up and kept answering calls from headhunters.

And unexpectedly, one of the lines I had cast in the water got a bite.

Because I held an active Kansas medical license, I caught the attention of a recruiter for an Ob/Gyn locum tenens opportunity at a different rural hospital in Kansas than the one I had negotiated with Dr. Arbus.

This facility had a dire need for an Ob/Gyn as one of the two physicians practicing there had moved, leaving a single doctor to manage a full service of patients. I offered to help in both the clinic and the hospital for one weekend a month, sticking to my preferred schedule of arriving on Thursday evening and traveling home on Sunday night.

This recruiter knew about my recent lack of hospital obstetrical experience, but she fought hard for me to be considered by the hospital's administration.

To my amazement, I was accepted for the position.

Hospital credentialing, Drug Enforcement Agency (DEA) licensure, medmal coverage, the costs of travel, and setting up my schedule were all handled by the recruiting company, which is typical of locums.

A few months later, I arrived for my first shift at a small rural hospital in the "middle of nowhere."

After finishing my first day in the clinic, I settled into the hotel room which would be my home away from home for the weekend.

I really didn't know what to expect once I was on call for the evening.

In preparation for the assignment, I sought advice from two of my closest colleagues regarding the basics of delivering a baby.

"You'll be fine. It's just like riding a bike!" they said.

Despite all my diligence in getting the job and the confidence I thought I had, I was nervous.

Was this a mistake?

On the second night of my assignment, the hotel phone rang at 3:00 am. An L&D nurse let me know a new patient had just arrived at the unit in active labor; she was 8 centimeters dilated. This was the patient's third baby, so I knew delivery would likely happen quickly.

I jumped out of bed and literally ran around the hotel room in circles, my heart racing as I realized, "This was it." I was going to deliver a baby after a thirteen-year hiatus from hospital obstetrics.

I rushed to the hospital in pitch-black darkness, trying not to speed on the rural road. Upon my arrival, the baby's head was visible each time the patient pushed. Trying to appear calm, I methodically reviewed the instruments that had been laid out on the delivery table and went through a mental checklist of the steps I would take to safely deliver the baby as well as what needed to be done following delivery. Clamping and cutting the umbilical cord, obtaining cord blood, delivering the placenta, repairing any lacerations, and ensuring that both the mother and baby were clinically stable. I realized the nurses were likely not aware that I hadn't been in L&D for over ten years and that this was my first L&D locum tenens assignment.

This realization only added to my anxiety.

Despite my calm exterior, I could feel my heart pounding in my chest and perspiration forming on my palms beneath the sterile gloves as my mind kept wandering to all the things that could go wrong, such as shoulder dystocia, sudden fetal bradycardia, and post-partum hemorrhage.

Thankfully, the delivery went smoothly, and the baby was a girl. It was the patient's third daughter, and I felt an immediate kinship with her. I was so endeared that the following morning while making hospital rounds, I asked a family member to take a photo of us.

I had not delivered a baby since 2004, when I left the group practice to return to academic medicine. Now, after so many seemingly insurmountable obstacles, over a period that seemed like ages, I had returned to the practice of obstetrics.

Thirteen years later.

I completed the long weekend assignments in rural Kansas that I had contracted for. When I was not needed at the hospital, I immersed myself in what the small town had to offer by visiting coffee shops and family restaurants, browsing bookshops and boutiques, venturing to the wetlands, and attending a local church service.

And thus, the stage was set for what would become my modus operandi when starting a new locum tenens assignment: Learn as much about the area's culture and people as possible to help me connect with the patients I was caring for and bond with the nursing staff.

When you're thrust into a new situation without knowing what to expect, it can be intimidating and unsettling. I discovered that by listening to the L&D nurses, I could find out more information regarding what was going on at that hospital and why they needed a locum tenens physician. Sometimes, the information I had been given by the recruiter was not the "whole story."

I viewed each locums opportunity as a possible permanent part-time position. It was difficult not to. When reflecting on my initial negotiations with the hospital in Kansas, it seemed logical to me that if there was a temporary need, there might be a permanent need. It became important to view these assignments as auditions.

Is this a place where I could see myself working long-term? What are my thoughts about the hospital culture, hospital administration, nursing staff, quality of ancillary services, and availability of consultants? Do I feel valued and respected by the patients and staff? Is it a good fit?

In parallel with my first Ob/Gyn assignment, I was negotiating for and was accepted for a weekend job in the panhandle region of Texas, which dovetailed with the final weekend I worked in rural Kansas.

Traveling to this new location was less complex, but I stipulated the same parameters regarding my preferred long weekend schedule.

The physician I would be covering for in Texas was in a similar situation to my previous gig. His partner had moved, and he was now the sole Ob/Gyn responsible for a full practice.

We had met each other a few years earlier when his office was further south in Texas. Dr. Daryl was an excellent obstetrician but did not have much experience with laparoscopic gynecologic surgery, so we decided to teach each other our skill sets.

I reviewed the gynecology surgery patients' charts remotely and gave my recommendations to Dr. Daryl regarding the workup and best surgical option. He would perform the appropriate pre-operative evaluation and schedule the case for a Friday when I was there. Additionally, he would schedule elective repeat Caesarean sections (C-sections) on the same Friday and give me a refresher by patiently guiding me through performing them.

For almost six months, I flew up to the panhandle every other weekend to work. I taught Dr. Daryl my technique for performing advanced laparoscopy cases, and he taught me his approach for elective repeat C-sections.

As I had done during my first travel assignment, I immersed myself in the community, established a good rapport with the hospital nurses, and enjoyed exploring the small town in the Texas panhandle.

During one of my assignments, a fierce blizzard blew into town and essentially shut it down. The hospital went on diversion, and I spent the weekend inside the hotel only being called for non-obstetrical emergencies as maternity patients were being sent to another hospital thirty miles away.

I took advantage of this downtime by exploring multiple job boards for locum tenens work, again broadening my search to include other states, even those where I didn't hold an active medical license. My travel stipulation was not to spend more than half a day getting to the location so that I could spend the front end of an assignment seeing patients in my office.

I found a contract position at a CAH in rural New Mexico. This position was not negotiated through a recruiting company but with the hospital administration directly. I applied, flew out for an interview with the administrative team, toured the hospital, and was accepted.

The job started shortly after the six-month assignment in Texas ended. My responsibilities included seeing patients in the clinic as well as taking call at the hospital. The opportunity was unique in that there were no permanent Ob/Gyns on the team. A midwife lived in town, and she was the hub in the wheel of care provided to the patients. I would be part of a group of four specialists and one family medicine physician who rotated on a set schedule to provide clinic and call coverage and back up the midwife. All the temps lived out of town; the CAH had not employed a permanent full-time Ob/Gyn physician for several years.

It was a novel experience, and I settled into traveling to the southern desert mountains of New Mexico each month, absorbing the culture, foods, scenery, and people of a place so different from where I practiced in Texas.

Given that this was a permanent position, I came to view my job in New Mexico as a "mini practice" and began to grow a patient base of my own and perform laparoscopy cases at the hospital, something that hadn't been done there for several years. I developed friendships outside of the work environment, and Wilson and I eventually purchased a small home there. It was nice not having to pack and unpack each month. We decorated our new house in a contemporary southwestern style, much different from the style of our home in Texas.

I was still able to manage my micro practice remotely while helping women in this underserved rural area of New Mexico. A direct two-hour flight between Houston and Albuquerque made the travel manageable, and I was able to see patients in my office the same day I traveled.

Over the past seven years, I've been fortunate to have worked at over fifteen hospitals in six states. For most of these assignments, I've been able to stick with the same parameters of starting the shift late in the week and providing coverage through the weekend in order to have a weekly presence in my practice. On occasion, I have extended my locum tenens coverage to longer periods of time.

The states I have worked in other than Texas, Kansas, and New Mexico include Hawaii, Oregon, and Idaho. Each location has been a learning experience career-wise and an adventure in terms of immersing myself in the local culture as a part of the workforce in the community.

Some of these positions were secured by working with head-hunters, and others were negotiated through direct contracts with the hospital system. There are advantages and disadvantages to each of these approaches.

Working with a recruiting company is helpful when first considering locums. Most hospital systems utilize more than one agency to search for locum tenens physicians when they need help. The recruiting agency assists the locum tenens candidates with credentialing, state licensure, negotiating a rate of pay, securing dates for assignments, airfare, lodging, and rental car expenses. All expenses incurred are covered by the recruiting company. The cost of meals is the responsibility of the locum tenens physician. However, at most of the hospitals I've worked at, there is a cafeteria or doctor's dining room with free access to meals. Some hotels offer free breakfasts, and I've stayed in lodging with a kitchen allowing for simple and affordable meal preparation. It is fun, however, to explore the local dining options when traveling. I have found the nurses in L&D to be quite forthcoming with restaurant recommendations as well as where the best coffee shop is located.

The main disadvantage of working with an agency is that the pay is generally lower than when you contract directly because the hospital must pay a commission to the "middleman". Most recruiting companies have several administrative assistants who will be involved in helping you with your assignment. It can sometimes be confusing when communicating with many individuals regarding one assignment. Over time, I have developed professional relationships with senior members of the teams at several of my favorite locum tenens companies.

Direct contracts with hospital systems are more challenging to secure but can help a locum tenens candidate be paid at a higher rate. Since fewer individuals are involved with the credentialing and onboarding process, it can proceed more smoothly.

The disadvantages of a direct contract with the hospital system are that the cost of licensure, medmal insurance, and travel expenses may be the responsibility of the locum tenens physician.

The position I have in New Mexico is a direct contract with the hospital system and comes with benefits such as retirement contributions, life insurance, health insurance, Health Savings Account (HSA) contributions, and a travel stipend. I have provided Ob/Gyn coverage for more than one hospital within the same system.

Compensation for locum tenens work is either as an independent contractor (1099) or an employer-employee W-2 arrangement. 1099 income isn't taxed upfront, so it's important to set aside a portion of your earnings for the federal income tax you will owe later.

Most recruiting companies will set up an independent contractor agreement between their corporation and the physician's business entity, such as an S-corporation (S-Corp) or Limited Liability Company (LLC). For the locum tenens work I do, the independent contractor 1099 agreement is between the recruiting company and S-Corp for my micro practice. Money earned from these assignments goes directly to my practice, untaxed.

W-2 agreements are between the individual physician and the hospital system when setting up a direct contract. That income is taxed and reported to the Internal Revenue Service (IRS) under your social security number.

When working multiple locum tenens assignments during the year, your tax bracket may change to your disadvantage. In general, the tax laws do not allow business deductions for W-2 income. I recommend discussing the tax advantages and disadvantages of the various contract options with your accountant.

While most of my experiences have been positive, there have been some that were unpleasant. For instance, a rooster's crows kept me awake all night at my lodging in a small central Texas town. On another occasion in Hawaii, there was inadequate backup for an obstetrical emergency that led to a poor clinical outcome. And for some of my first assignments, I received very low pay. But overall, the nurses and ancillary staff have been welcoming and helpful, and most importantly, the patients are appreciative of a physician coming to help.

I never dreamed that after leaving obstetrics almost twenty years ago, I would return to the specialty and experience such a rich diversity of job opportunities. The professional fulfillment I achieved was never expected. By working at different hospital systems and embracing the local cultures of so many diverse regions of our country, I have become a better physician. Locum tenens became my mission work, and I strongly encourage all physicians to consider this as a viable possibility.

My job at the CAH in New Mexico, where I negotiated my first direct locums contract over six years ago, became my major source of income as my micro practice was recovering from the pandemic. I continue to work there sporadically as well as sub at other hospital systems and have become more selective regarding which assignments I choose. I base my decision on the compensation offered, the presence of a safe hospital culture, and its proximity to my home in Texas.

- *By working with a recruiting company, the administrative requirements and negotiations are handled by a third party*
- *The recruiting company will arrange and pay for the costs of licensure and travel*
- *There can be multiple parties involved when working with a recruiting company leading to complex communication*
- *By directly negotiating a contract with a hospital system, a higher rate of pay can be achieved*
- *Independent contractor jobs are reported as 1099 income to the IRS and are not taxed*
- *Employer-employee contracts are reported as W-2 income to the IRS and are subject to the usual taxation*

PLASMAPHERESIS WORK AND THE PANDEMIC

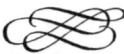

*S*hortly after launching my micro practice, I secured a small business loan to help with overhead expenses as I was transitioning from the MSO to new individual contracts with payors.

My friend Mary had decided to pursue a law degree shortly before I started the business school program. She worked side gigs to help with her tuition and graciously kept sending me opportunities that she thought I might be interested in.

One of these prospects was to become a medical director for a plasmapheresis company. It was a 1099 position.

At first, I was skeptical as I had an unhealthy bias toward the plasma donation industry. I remember my youngest daughter Maggie calling me when she was in college, asking what I thought about her donating plasma twice a week for extra money. At the time, I was horrified. Weren't these places where people with substance abuse issues went to get money to support their habits? Were they clean? Safe? My answer to Maggie was an emphatic "No!"

Mary had been working as a medical director for the plasmapheresis industry for a few years, so was able to give me details of the job. The position was non-clinical and required an on-site commitment at the plasma center of four hours each week per Food and Drug

Administration (FDA) regulations. This was doable given I was seeing patients in my office two and a half days each week and could easily add another half day plus commute time to a plasmapheresis center. Once I heard more about the role from Mary, I decided to pursue it.

As Center Medical Director (CMD), I was part of the Medical Operations Team and was responsible for oversight of the staff who screened potential donors as well as handling any health issues related to the donation process. Other responsibilities included working with the Quality Team, giving lectures at monthly meetings, and being available during normal business hours for any questions regarding donor suitability or abnormal screening results.

I was also the Laboratory Director (LD), which required both Commission on Laboratory Accreditation (COLA) training and a Clinical Laboratory Improvement Amendments (CLIA) license, which was paid for by the company. As LD, I was responsible for signing off on everyone in the center who performed moderate-complexity testing, as well as reviewing the standards for calibrating the instruments.

I began working at several centers in the Houston area and discovered that people from all walks of life come to donate plasma. The donors receive a debit card that can be used to buy groceries or pay utility bills. The facilities are very clean, well-run, and operate under strict federal guidelines.

My preconception was incorrect.

When the COVID-19 pandemic hit, like so many other practices and businesses, my patient volume took a deep dive. The Governor of Texas shut down businesses for two months. In other states, the restrictions were more severe. Elective surgeries couldn't be performed. Patients were afraid to come to their physicians' offices due to concerns regarding becoming infected with the virus.

I applied for and received an emergency loan offered through the federal government and stepped up my side gig game.

One of the CMDs working for the plasmapheresis company received an internal promotion during this time. She asked me if I would cover her centers until full-time replacements could be found. Given I had a lot more time on my hands, coupled with the uncertainty regarding when or if life would return to normal, I agreed to help.

I started traveling to four different centers each week, one of them as far away as one hundred miles. The hourly pay was good, and I was also reimbursed for mileage. This compensation helped with my overhead expenses at a time when my practice volume had declined by more than fifty percent.

The direct contract locums position I held in New Mexico emerged as my primary source of income. Thankfully, there were also benefits associated with this job, as previously mentioned. I began to increase the number of days each month that I traveled to New Mexico, along with running my micro practice and working as a CMD for the plasma centers. I also added other weekend locum tenens jobs that were within half a day's driving distance from home.

Enduring the effects of COVID-19 on daily life was stressful, and in 2021, I received heartbreaking news that my mother had been diagnosed with advanced uterine cancer. She lived over three hours away, and when I wasn't working, I would travel to see her as much as possible. We spoke on the phone every day.

For two years, Mom fought this terrible disease and coped with complex surgery, chemotherapy, and radiation without complaining. Her "stiff upper lip" approach to life and joyful demeanor were, and continue to be, such an inspiration to me.

She wasn't in remission for very long, and it became my responsibility to tell Mom and Dad that she was terminal. Her oncologist offered her more chemotherapy even though the prognosis was poor and the potential side effects were harsh. It was an excruciatingly difficult conversation to have with my parents. As the eldest daughter, I was now one of my mother's caregivers who just happened to be a physician with experience working at a cancer center.

My siblings and I arranged home hospice care per Mom's wishes. I took some time off to spend a few days with her once she was home. Our extended family took shifts at my parents' apartment to help Dad administer Mom's medications and care for her. I learned a lot about what services are covered by Medicare and supplemental insurance policies for hospice patients and how essential it is to have a family member as your advocate when terminally ill.

On the last day I was there, I kissed her gently and whispered, "I love you, Mom. I'll see you on Wednesday."

She died at home a few days later before I could return.

I miss her.

I'm grateful that I created a career portfolio and became autonomous with my micro practice, as it enabled me to be there for my mother and family during that grievous time.

EXPERT WITNESS WORK

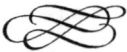

This side gig is one of my favorites. I enjoy sleuthing through medical records, researching current standards of care related to the case I'm reviewing, and interacting with attorneys. I feel that by participating in the medicolegal process, I am a better physician. I have worked for both defense and plaintiff's attorneys. I have written medical file reports, been deposed, and testified in court.

The advantages of working as a medical expert witness include:

1. Set your own schedule
2. Intellectually challenging
3. High rate of pay
4. 1099 compensation
5. Opportunity to help pursue justice for either the injured patient or the accused physician
6. Learning about the laws regarding medical negligence (tort) in various states

The disadvantages of working as a medical expert witness include:

1. Get labeled as a "gun for hire"

2. Have your written words revised by counsel to strengthen their case
3. Testify against another physician

Should you decide to pursue this opportunity, I recommend going to the TASA website (tasanet.com) to create a listing as well as explore the biographies of expert witnesses listed in your field. Networking on LinkedIn is also wise. There are online courses and podcasts of physicians who coach prospective expert witnesses.

A physician who works in this field should be actively practicing medicine and not semi or fully retired from clinical practice.

TELEMEDICINE

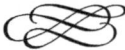

*D*uring the COVID-19 pandemic, organizations were forced to pivot to different models of delivering care to maintain patient and worker safety from potential exposure to the virus. Although the concept of providing medical care virtually via synchronous or asynchronous platforms has been in existence for many years, this technology exploded in early 2020.

Telemedicine offers a wide variety of services, including care for patients across a broad spectrum of specialties including primary care, psychiatry, weight loss, dermatology, and authorization of medical marijuana cards. Areas of women's health infiltrated by tele-health companies include menopause symptoms, contraception, and urinary tract infections.

Many telemedicine businesses are start-ups. One of the goals of these companies is to garner enough profit via virtual visits to make them attractive to investors. This means the business may fold if not bought out, potentially putting a physician's job in jeopardy.

The advantages of working for a telemedicine company include:

1. Set your own schedule

2. Ability to blend a few remote visits each day with running your own practice or working at other jobs
3. Streamlined patient assessment and treatment plans according to algorithms established by the company

The disadvantages of working for a telemedicine company include:

1. Low rate of pay
2. Volume driven
3. Liability issues related to relying on patients' self-reported data such as weight and blood pressure given that no objective data is collected
4. Potential lack of job security when working for a start-up company
5. Multiple state licensures required
6. Learning a non-traditional (usually homegrown) EHR

If pursuing a side gig in this industry appeals to you, I recommend the following:

1. Search major job boards as well as those specific to telemedicine companies
2. Network on LinkedIn with physicians and administrators who are working for specific telehealth organizations
3. Obtain the Interstate Medical Licensure Compact (IMLC)

Once you've got your foot in the door:

1. During contract negotiations, be sure to stipulate your weekly availability as well as whether you will be responsible for the cost of medmal coverage and state licensing
2. Telemedicine companies pay either per patient encounter

or by the hour. Ask whether you'll be compensated if a patient is a "no show"

3. Training on the platform's EHR should be paid
4. Ask whether you'll be responsible for supervising nurse practitioners

CONCLUSION: WHERE I AM NOW

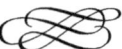

*F*ollowing the pandemic recovery, my surgical volume did not rebound as I had hoped. In addition, reimbursements for the surgeries I performed continued to decline. Despite obtaining appropriate prior authorization approval from payors, payment for surgery was sometimes denied after the procedure had been performed, or a patient's out-of-pocket costs exceeded what was estimated, and she owed a balance.

For several years, I have been reading about the Direct Primary Care (DPC) movement. Two of my closest friends who own internal medicine and neurology practices have successfully transitioned away from the traditional insurance-based model and are now cash-based. When I initially began to research this option for my micro practice, I was hesitant to move forward as this would mean giving up being in the operating room, a passion of mine since residency.

Two years ago, my employees and I implemented a transparent structure of self-pay prices. This included posting a menu of services offered along with their cost on my website. We had conducted a market survey, and our prices were set within an affordable range for the women we care for.

Since implementing this change, a steady *uptick* in the number of women booking appointments as self-pay patients has occurred. These patients are uninsured, underinsured, or insured by plans outside my network.

In mid-2024, after gauging the response of patients to a cash-based practice, I felt I had grown a large enough patient base to support implementing that business model. This meant dropping insurance contracts completely.

It was time. After two years of offering a hybrid practice model that combined revenues from self-pay patients with those covered by in-network payor contracts, I was ready to transition completely to a cash-based micro practice. The income from the independent contractor jobs I had curated would provide financial stability during this time.

We sent letters to all the insurance companies giving them six months' notice that I was going out of network. Additionally, all active patients were informed of this decision through the EHR as well as in person at the time of their office visits. Because opting out of Medicare can be a laborious process, I elected to maintain my contract with traditional Medicare.

I have been overwhelmed by the support of most of my patients. I would estimate that 80 percent of my patients have decided to keep me as their doctor.

Interestingly, the patients who have not been receptive are those with higher financial means or are covered by more desirable insurance plans.

Surprisingly, new patients are booking appointments with me *specifically* because I don't deal with insurance anymore. I feel this is because we offer same-day or next-day appointments, which patients without insurance often don't have access to. I also feel patients respect and appreciate my decision to work directly for them rather than be beholden to corporate guidelines.

I continue to work independent contractor jobs linked to my micro practice S-Corp. As discussed before, this money goes into my practice account to help with office overhead expenses. My goal is to be completely "in the black," with all debts incurred during the pandemic paid off by the end of 2025.

I have narrowed my focus to only those side gigs that bring me joy and allow me to best utilize my professional strengths and experiences. My hope is that with more time, I will be able to cut back on these extra jobs, stop working more than forty hours a week between all my professional obligations, and transition to a lighter schedule as I prepare for semi-retirement.

Through networking on social media and listening to podcasts, I have a grasp of the current climate for private practitioners in our increasingly complex healthcare system, and I am excited to embark on this next journey in my career.

For me, blending the ownership of a micro practice with side gigs has propelled me past feelings of disillusionment. By continuing to explore new opportunities, my professional life remains interesting and challenging. I feel that by creating a diverse career portfolio, a physician's brain remains stimulated, avoiding the burnout that can occur when working within a system that promotes a "hamster on the wheel" mentality. I'm at the point in my career where if I try something new and don't fully enjoy it, I stop doing it.

There have been bumps in the road. Countless days of tears, feeling physically and emotionally exhausted, and wanting to give up. But I have pressed on. As I enter a phase of life when so many of my friends, either physicians or in other careers, are retiring, I plan to continue working.

Wilson and I have three grandsons, and I want to be able to spend as much time with them as possible, as well as with our aging parents, who are in their 90s. We look forward to more sailing as our boat has been lonely. As long as I can spend time with family, care for my patients and my two dedicated employees, stay healthy, and enjoy our hobbies, I intend to continue this plan for as long as possible.

I also want to help other physicians feel empowered in our current healthcare system. By recognizing the constraints that comprise our corporatized medicine structure, we can learn how to function more positively and with more satisfaction.

Private equity is the new albatross around the necks of those who practice in the United States. If there was ever a time when profit came before patient care, it is now.

I am calling on my readers to re-align themselves with their core values of why they entered medical school in the first place and to separate themselves as much as possible from the influences of investment groups and large corporations. This means diverting yourself from those decisions that solely lead to monetary gain and instead, finding an avenue through which you can allow access for all to the skill set you have, regardless of a patient's ability to pay.

There is no playbook for success, but I hope the story of my career journey over the past three decades will embolden others to look outside the box, be entrepreneurial, and remain in charge of how and where they choose to practice medicine.

By creating a "career portfolio", physicians can maintain enthusiasm when things go well and take a pause when things don't.

Our healthcare system is fractured. We *can* fix it.

If more physicians become autonomous, maybe those who are making our professional lives so miserable will realize that there can be no healthcare without doctors. Then we'll be able to deliver high-quality care to our patients without sacrificing our own physical, mental, and financial health.

Be well.

RESOURCES

Books

1. Wilner, AN. (2018). *The Locum Life: A Physician's Guide to Locum Tenens*. Lulu Publishing Services.
2. Blaine, D. (2024). *The WriteR Stuff: Step-By-Step Guide to Self-Publishing and Worldwide Distribution*. Very Indie Press.

Articles

3. (2024). aamc.org. *2024 Facts: Applicants and Matriculants Data.* https://www.aamc.org/data-reports/students-residents/data/facts-applicants-and-matriculants
4. Darves, B. (2024, August 9). nejmcareercenter.org. *Physicians' Career Priorities and Expectations Undergoing Shifts.* https://resources.nejmcareercenter.org/article/physicians-career-priorities-and-expectations-undergoing-shifts/
5. Miller, D. (2023, November 8). whitecoatinvestor.com. *A Step-by-Step Guide to Starting a Medical Practice.* https://www.whitecoatinvestor.com/start-medical-practice/
6. Gibbons, M. (2024, December 25). kevinmd.com. *Rethinking shift work: Why "job sharing" is the key to happier, healthier doctors.* https://kevinmd.com/2024/12/rethinking-shift-work-why-job-sharing-is-the-key-to-happier-healthier-doctors.html
7. Rhodes, H. (2022, September 15). kevinmd.com. *Don't give up on private practice just yet.* https://kevinmd.com/2022/09/dont-give-up-on-private-practice-just-yet.html
8. (2018). comptroller.texas.com. *A Storm to Remember: Hurricane Harvey and the Texas Economy.* https://comptroller.texas.gov/economy/fiscal-notes/archive/2018/special-edition/impact.php
9. (2023, November 17), thecommonwealthfund.org. *Private Equity's Role in Healthcare.* https://www.commonwealthfund.org/publications/explainer/2023/nov/private-equity-role-health-care

Websites

10. American Association for Physician Leadership. https://www.physicianleaders.org
11. KSTAR Physician Resources. https://architexas.org/programs/kstar-physician/index.html
12. The TASA Group. https://www.tasanet.com

13. Doctor's Crossing. https://doctorscrossing.com
14. NonClinical Physicians https://nonclinicalphysicians.com/
15. All Things Writing. https://allthingswriting.com
16. Starting a Micropractice: A Physician's Guide. https://www.physiciansidegigs.com/starting-a-micropractice

ACKNOWLEDGMENTS

I have so many people to thank for where I am today.

My husband, parents, daughters, extended family and friends, two dedicated employees, my patients, countless co-workers, nurses, mentors, and my faith.

Thank you to my writing coach, Debra Blaine, who inspired me to continue telling my story even when I was ready to give up.

I realize that I possess a driven personality and never experienced significant adversity when growing up. My parents instilled in me the importance of working hard and finishing the job while having fun along the way.

I have also been the recipient of opportunities that I didn't pursue and realize that not everyone is so fortunate.

I miss Mom. Although she may not have always agreed with my decisions, she was consistently supportive and understanding. We became close friends later in life.

I keep a framed photograph of Mom in my New Mexico home. How I wish she could have come out for a visit during one of my shifts there as I feel she would have loved it.

In my heart, I know she is there. Supporting me, encouraging me, and living inside me as I drive to the hospital on those cool, dark New Mexico nights.

To deliver a baby.

ABOUT THE AUTHOR

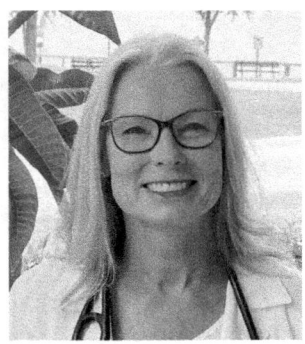

Dr. Helen Rhodes is an obstetrician-gynecologist currently practicing in coastal Texas and the desert mountains of New Mexico. She is passionate about helping others recognize when it's time to pivot and enjoys sharing her insight through writing and mentoring. Dr. Rhodes is an advocate for the preservation of physician autonomy and career reinvention. In her spare time, she enjoys traveling, water sports, hiking, gardening, baking, and spending time with her growing extended family.

The Power to Pivot is Dr. Rhodes's debut book, offering guidance and inspiration for physicians seeking clarity, renewed purpose, and balance in their careers. She may be reached at drhelenrhodes@gmail.com.